Tight Hip Flexors

The Ultimate Cure to Unlock Tight Hip, Twisted core, Sore Shoulders & Lower back Pain with Exercises

Ray Randy

Copyright

Disclaimer & Statement of Rights

TABLE OF CONTENTS

INTRODUCTION 1

ANATOMY OF THE HIP FLEXORS 5

ABOUT PSOAS 12

FIGHT OR FLIGHT MUSCLE FOR SURVIVAL 19

HOW SITTING TOO MUCH CAN DESTROY YOUR HEALTH 23

SITTING AND YOUR SEX LIFE 28

EMOTIONAL EFFECTS OF TIGHT PSOAS 32

ENHANCE POWER TO INCREASE PERFORMANCE 34

EFFECTS OF TIGHT HIPS ON WEIGHT 44

EFFECTS OF WEAK PSOAS MUSCLES ON EMOTION AND ENERGY 53

STRETCHING   58

STATIC STRETCHING, NOT THE ONLY ANSWER   73

THE POWERFUL HIP FLEXORS DIET   78

HIP FLEXOR STRETCHES FOR ELDERS   97

CONCLUSION   109

INTRODUCTION

Most people will be walking around, not knowing that they are having tight hip flexors.

Do you know that hip flexors are the parts of the body responsible for most movements, such as stability and energetic movements that include kicking? All these movements play an essential role in most of our daily activities. Therefore if they get tight, they will exhibit lots of health issues. The hip flexors consist of two muscles-the psoas and the iliacus.

Anatomically, the psoas is attached to the lower back, and it is placed at the top of the thigh bone. The iliacus is attached to the hip bone and placed at the top of the thigh bone. These two muscles, in combination, will form iliopsoas muscle. The iliopsoas is a long muscle, though not pliable, and they are involved in many small and large movements.

The most challenging adverse effects of tight hips are back pain. It has been discovered that back pain affects many people, and surprisingly most of them do not know why they are experiencing such pain. The hip flexor is attached to the lower back, and if the setting is tight, it will pull the lower back forward. This condition will put the person into lordosis, though some people are known to have an enormous curve in the lower back, it can be severe pain for others. When going into lordosis, it put lots of pressure on the lower back, and will also put more pressure on the intervertebral discs.

Tight hip flexor pain can be seen in most activities in the core, back, and upper legs that require power. Most often, athletes experience tight hip flexors when they are performing weighted lifts such as deadlifts and squats. When the flexor muscles are tight, they tend to prevent pelvis, spine, and hip complex from proper alignment.

This improper alignment may lead to bottom switching off. The psoas and glute are antagonists, meaning that when one is working, the other is relaxing. So invariably, while the glute is relaxing, the hip flexor is working. This may result in having back issues, as the lower back muscles will be doing the work that the bottom should be doing. That means extra work on the muscles will put additional strain and will lead to been injured.

Unlocking tight hip flexors and tension is not as easy as some people may claim. Relieving tight hip flexors requires some specific exercises that are targeted at the deep tissues of the body's core. Some of these exercises require commitments that some people may deem uncomfortable.

Sitting all day like a desk job, car travel, or long flights have been known to be the major cause of tight hip flexors. It has been discovered that the more time we spend sitting, the more shortened the iliopsoas. And the shorter the muscle, the shorter the stride becomes. This shortness will l imbalance, and there will be a compensation to the imbalance. This will lead to injury in the muscles that are responsible for our movements.

The stretches exercise illustrated in this guide will help in unlocking your tight hip flexors, and you will be able to experience the ability to move legs in a full range of motion. Other benefits include a longer running stride, comfortable seating path such as squats, jumping, biking, driving, dancing, hiking, and host of others.

ANATOMY OF THE HIP FLEXORS

We are unique creatures. However, there is an exception to this statement as our physical bodies were designed differently. Without considering traits such as skin, weight, colour, look and height, the entire population looks and functions the same with the aid of the human body. There is no doubt that the human body is very complex and can be difficult to understand when we go into the study of biomechanics and its effects on the whole human body.

The basic is that when the arm has been flexed, the biceps bracii will be shortened or contracted. This is due to the basic anatomy and physiology, but if we are to consider the natural response of the body to curling of the arm things will get more complicated. Now let's check the exact fixator muscles, antagonist, agonist, and synergist.

Understanding the basic workings of the complexity of the human body takes years of research, and even at that level, there are still many mysteries uncovered about the human body. There are some parts of the human body that have a more significant impact on the human body than other parts—putting into consideration arms, hips or shoulders. We could see that arms were simple in designs and functions and will have little impact on the overall state of the body comparing to others like hips and shoulders.

No doubt that shoulders are more complex in

the design and functions, but this book will focus on the hips. The hips are known to be the most crucial region of the body, and this book will discuss in details the ultimate benefits of having healthy and good hip flexors.

Human anatomy made us understand that it is challenging to function appropriately if the hips are not in a good state. Hips have a significant impact on virtually everything we do from sitting to standing, twisting, reaching, bending, stepping, walking and many other physical activities.

It is still possible to stand or sit if you are having a broken arm, or torn rotator cuff, but can it be possible with a fractured hip or torn hip flexor; No. The hips cater for ultimate power and life's movement. The basic anatomy of hips is complex, but we will paint a clear picture of it for better understanding.

Bone structure:

Three bones in the pelvis of the adults would be fused into acetabulum or hipbone that formed part of the hip region. The hip joint known scientifically as acetabulofemora is the joint in between acetabulum and femur of the pelvis. Its main objective is to support the weight of the body while standing (static), and walking or running (position).

The hip joints do more function in retaining balance. The hips do no wonder at the inclination angle, which happens to be the most crucial element of the human body.

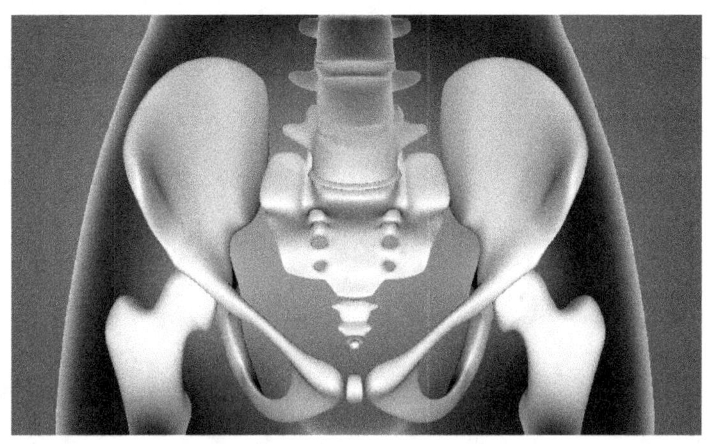

Hip flexors

The hip part of the body composed of over 15 muscles that are very important in the function of the hips and the surrounding bones. The hip region is divided into 4 muscle groups.

The gluteal group: This group is the major contributor to hip extension.

The lateral rotator group: This group is in charge of lateral rotation of the hips.

The abductor/adductor group: This group is in control of the inward and outward movement of the femur.

The iliopsoas group: This group is responsible for hip flexion.

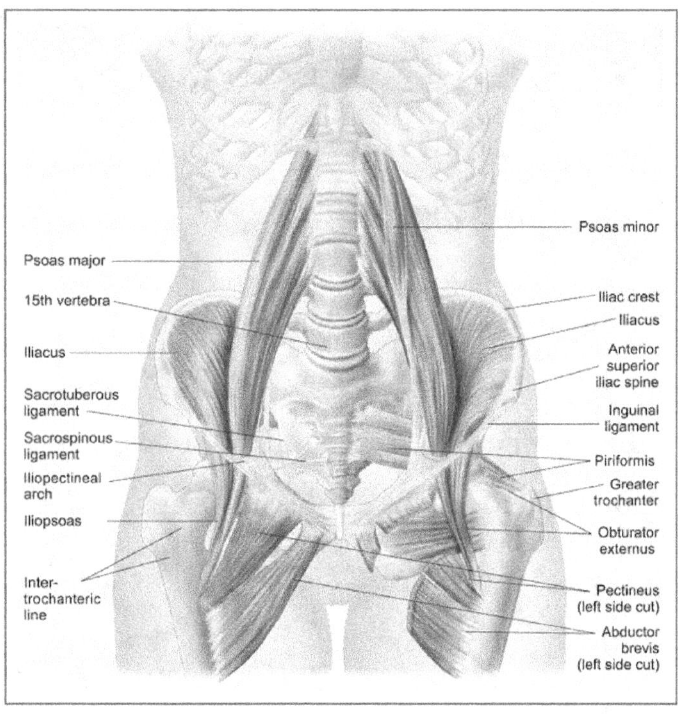

As discussed earlier that each of this group is responsible for certain roles of the hips. However, the muscles are not meant only for precise movements. Every muscle group in the

above groups will act as the fixator muscles, antagonist, agonist, and synergist. For all the group muscles to work appropriately as was designed, some things must come into place for them to function correctly.

All these groups' muscles have their certain functions there a particular group known as iliopsoas has more responsibility than others.

ABOUT PSOAS

The psoas muscles are situated deep in the hip and are the most popular muscles when it comes to fitness. Many books, articles, videos have shown how it can be rehab videos, therapy and yoga. They all claimed it to be a vital factor for emotional, physical and spiritual well-being.

As discussed earlier, the psoas is one of the 4 groups known as the iliopsoas group. The psoas is a two-part muscle group made up of the iliacus and psoas. That's what made up the term iliopsoas. There are two types of the psoas and are the psoas major and psoas minor, but whenever psoas muscle is being mentioned, it is the psoas major that is being referenced. The reason has been that the function of psoas minor is minimal and is known to be a weak mover.

It is known that all iliopsoas group muscles work in harmony together, but iliacus is not as crucial as the psoas. Not like the psoas, the iliacus is within the hip and is responsible partially for flexing the hip and bending. However, the psoas is the main mover in the flexing and bending of the body.

The main reason the psoas is so popular is that it has many significant roles. Such roles include the structural level where it is responsible for the stabilizing of the spine and flexing of the hip. It also helps in the rotation of the femur outward and moving it to midlife (adducting). Another significant responsibility of the psoas is that it helps in connecting the legs to the spine.

Meaning anything you do with your legs can affect the spine without thinking about or feeling it.

The psoas is situated at the deep within the anterior hip joint and lower spine. The psoas major has been known to work independently and yet together as a team. They are attached to the side and toward the front of the 12th thoracic vertebrae and can be found on each lumbar vertebrae.

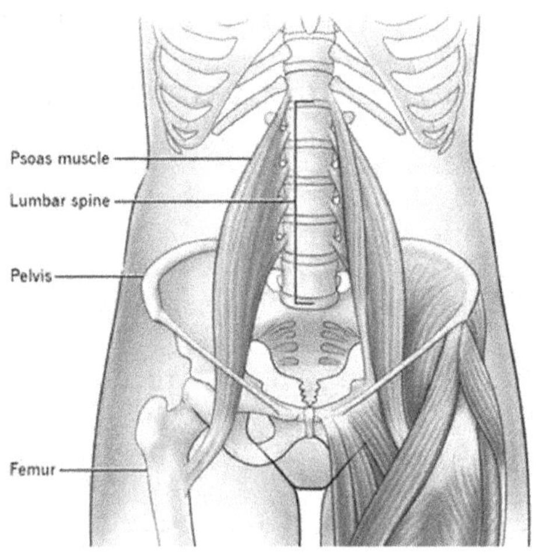

The psoas move through the pelvis without been attached to the bone, and they are inserted along with the iliacus in a tendon on top of the femur. Anatomically, the psoas is structured in such a way to provide a critical component for optimal postural alignment and overall health. The psoas is known to be the only muscle in the body that links the lower body and upper body and is critical in extending to the nerve complex and energy systems that are in the center of the body.

Another responsibility of the psoas is to give diagonal support via the trunk, thereby creating a shelf for the organs of the abdominal region. Whenever you are walking the psoas will moves freely and links with a released diaphragm to be able to maintain a stable and secured spine, also blood vessels, organs, and nerves of the trunk. A perfect psoas will give a delicate but critical connection between the legs and the upper body.

When the psoas is in excellent condition, it is expected to guide the transfer of weight from the trunk to the legs and be able to acts as a pathway to guide the flow of subtle energies. It is expected of psoas when in perfect condition to function like the tie-down of a tent that will stabilize the spine. So it is expected of it to support the foundation so as not to be compromised.

The psoas is also one of the significant contributors to the protection of the spine by making sure that the spine stabilizes the skeleton. Don't forget that psoas has the ability to tighten and release independently at any of its joints attachments. This will make it to be able to counterbalance the structure that is an imbalance in many ways.

In a situation where the psoas always contracts to correct the skeletal instability, the muscle may be shortened eventually and lose its flexibility and integrity. And once the original structure of the psoas has been changed, the body may quickly enter a defect condition.

Once the psoas is chronically shortened, some adverse conditions will rear their ugly heads if not attended to appropriately. This condition will make other muscles want to compensate for the loss of structural reliability. This will may hip to start tilting forward, changing the distances of some joints and the structures of bones, and femurs would want to compact into the hip sockets. To compensate for this structural imbalance, the upper thigh muscles (quadriceps) will become overdeveloped and may lead to lower back pain and knee pain.

To prevent the psoas imbalance in recent as a result of sedentary life that's why there is over-emphasis on the use of comfortable chairs, hip pain, sitting too much, and psoas related lower knee and back pain. Even active athletes also suffer from psoas imbalance and pain if they don't monitor the kind of activity they are engaged.

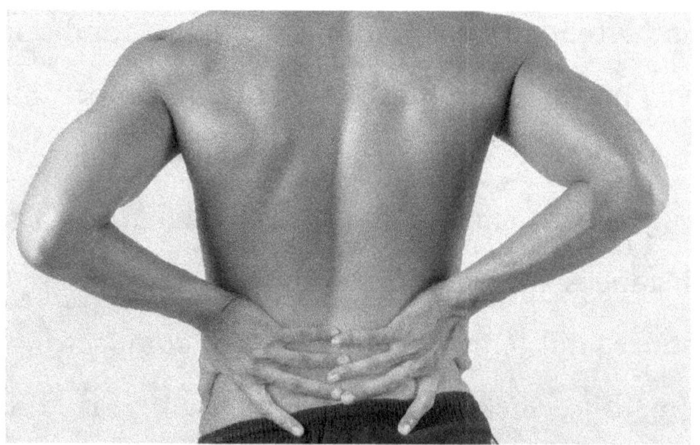

FIGHT OR FLIGHT MUSCLE FOR SURVIVAL

We have discussed psoas, what is SNS?

SNS is the Sympathetic Nervous System. SNS is a nervous system in the body that is essential for survival. SNS is one of the primary divisions of the autonomic nervous system; the other method is known as the parasympathetic nervous system.

Survival instinct has been with human body since the beginning. All animals and even some plant possess some mechanisms in them to help increase the survival instinct. Though modern survival may not be like that of our ancestors, some specific components in the human body remain unchanged when it comes to survival, and this includes SNS.

This survival system caters for two primary purposes. First, it aids the homeostasis within the body; keeping the body balanced.

SNS is also the main factor in the fight or flight response. This kind of response is what you experience whenever there is a dangerous situation.

What's the connection between SNS and psoas muscle?

The response triggered by the sympathetic nervous system will activate the iliopsoas muscles directly. Whether you jump out of the way, curl into a ball, you counter-attack, the response is primarily controlled by SNS. Its survival instinct.

This response of either fight or flight starts from the brain stem that connects to the spinal cord. The brain stem is in controlling the autonomic functions such as heart rate, breathing, and the fight or flight response. It also controls other social behaviours that may want to affect survival, like mating and dominance.

It is the fight or flight response that interacts directly with the iliopsoas muscles. When faced with sudden danger, the iliopsoas muscles will respond by bringing the two ends of your spinal cord together.

Iliopsoas muscles also help in the rolling body into a ball when curling into a fetal position. This intuitive response will assist in protecting the face and other vital organs. This is a natural response to danger that is triggered by the sympathetic nervous system and done by the iliopsoas muscles.

Have you found yourself in a dangerous situation where you kick or jump? This is also a response that activates the iliopsoas muscles.

There is a strong relationship between psoas muscles and the sympathetic nervous system. If this cordial relationship is put into danger, the natural ability to react to a threat will be threatened.

HOW SITTING TOO MUCH CAN DESTROY YOUR HEALTH

As discussed previously, the iliopsoas is very critical for survival, and attention must be paid on how to treat the related muscles in the body. It has been discovered that one of the biggest causes (but can be controlled) of tightness and imbalance of the hip is excess sitting. There are have been several news headlines that stated that sitting is more dangerous than smoking. That those set of people that sit too much are likely to die at an early age than those who don't sit too much.

If you are among those who sit all day or you are the type that drives during a good portion of the day, the following information is for your consumption.

It doesn't matter what sort of work you are doing while sitting too long in a chair; sitting in a stiff chair on a long-distance, writing a term paper, typing a lengthy business contract, writing your book, or hauling goods across the country. There is one thing that is common to occur to all the above categories, they are all placing their bodies in an unfavourable position, and this will lead to the body getting stiff.

This stiffness is generated from the backward tilt of the hips. While you decide to get up from the sitting all day to get work out to ease the pressure out from the legs, you only exacerbate the same pattern of sitting with many other exercises. This is not to say that you should avoid going to the gym, but the fact remains that the regular crunches and sit-ups will not help your hips. So it is crucial to keep the legs and glutes healthy. But be aware that much of flexion of the hip will limit the range of motion in the hips and may cause lower back and the knees to carry all the pressure.

Know that if you constantly sit in a chair for a long period, on a regular basis, your muscles may be shortened in length and it may be challenging to stand up straight.

If this tension is accumulated within the spine and hips, the muscles will become too tight, and it may be difficult to sleep on your stomach when lying down.

The same thing will also happen to your back and hamstrings, but its only back and knees that will be affected, which will result in deep pain in the groin and hip region. Then there will be deep ache in the stomach and follow by lower back pain that persists. This is an adverse effect of sitting too much.

With this condition, is it advisable to stop going to work or school to avoid sitting for too long?

But it is possible to change the sitting position and add routine exercises that can alleviate the situation. Businesses are even becoming aware of this condition, no wonder they are providing standing desks in the workplace, and walking breaks have been encouraged. But a fact must be established here, standing all day will not solve the problem on the ground as the damage has been done for years. Serious steps must be taken to correct the imbalances that have taken over.

Spending too much time in the chair in a flexed

position with a lack of no movement throughout the day will lead to tight iliopsoas muscles.

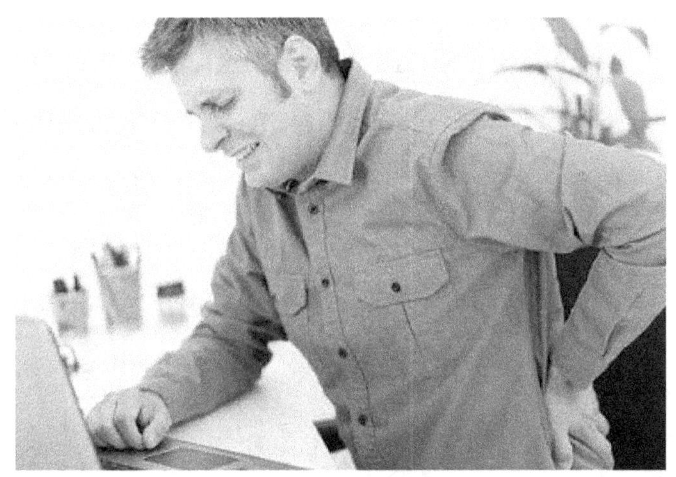

SITTING AND YOUR SEX LIFE

We all aware that the more active we are, the healthier, but why would sitting all day affect sex life? If sitting too much will affect ones healthy, what does the psoas have to do with sex? No doubt that sex is wonderful and who wouldn't want to enjoy it to the fullest. But truth be told, sitting all day will affect your sex life.

Let's consider these two cases: you have been on your feet all day, moving from one point to another, making sure that things are accomplished, getting a little sweat from the physical activity. These activities make you exhausted at the end of the day, and you have a sense of completion.

Another case is you have been sitting for over 8 hours with little movement, exhausted at the end. The difference is instead of a feeling sense of completion of hard work, but the feeling is horrible. Don't forget that body loves to move, and sex is also a movement. However, remember that not all movement is beneficial to the body.

As discussed earlier, sitting too much will lead to tightness in the psoas that causes stiffness throughout the body. In as much that psoas is responsible for good health and bad health, it is vital to take care of this region of the body.

Pain that may occur in the lower and middle back as well as abdominal or hips may lead to shallow breathing and difficulty in the movement of the hips. This has to do with how somebody functions will not be able to happen smoothly from limitation and restriction of muscles and organs. Not only will this pain affect sexual performance but also in the way the body reacts to pain as a threat. It will move the body from the state of pleasure to a state of panic.

When the psoas is tight as a result of sitting all day, the hips will become fixed in a position that is forward thrust. This position will cause the pelvis and legs to rotate. The forward tilt position will make the hip socket become compress leading to shifting and pulling of tendons, joints, and muscles been pulled from the lower back. This pulling on the lower back will reduce the flow and circulation of blood which will lead to delayed nerve response to the hips; thereby leading to non-performance on your sexual life.

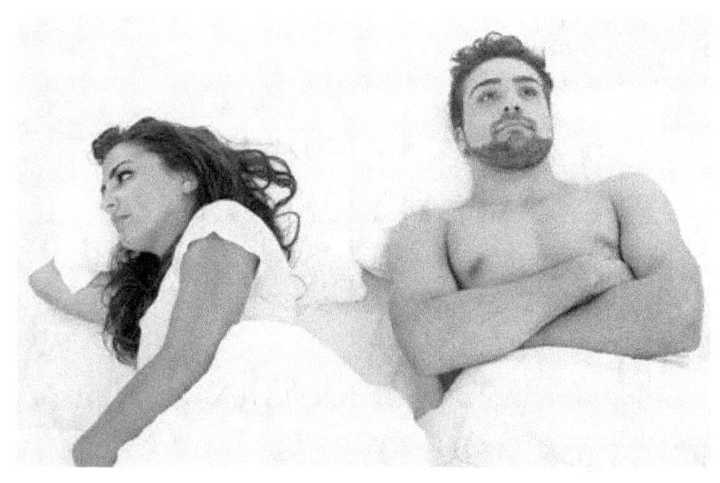

EMOTIONAL EFFECTS OF TIGHT PSOAS

We all aware that emotions are one of the major contributors to the current state of sex life.

Previously we discussed fight or flight response, the SNS, and the psoas. All these factors have a great impact on emotions and mental state that directly affect sexual life.

The fight or flight response increase or reduce your sexual appetite. Also, if you have a tight psoas muscle, signals will be sent from the brain to the body that danger is about to happen. These signals will automatically trigger responses in the body that may lead to overexertion of the adrenal glands and may weaken the body's natural immune response to stress.

Be aware that if you are having constant tight and overworked psoas, the body will face emotional and physical roadblock stress that will force the brain to continually send warning signals to all the body system that include the reproductive system.

Don't ever think that a tight psoas is just a physical limitation; it's also an emotional limitation.

Remember that hips are the main mover during sex, and it is reasonable to make the hips lose and flexible to be able to have dynamic sex.

ENHANCE POWER TO INCREASE PERFORMANCE

It is important that you build the strength of the hips flexors if you want to reach peak performance. As this is critical for athletes. It doesn't matter the kind of sport, and performance is significant as it comes down to power and they rely on strong, healthy hips.

Healthy hips are important if you are to function properly. As athletes required a proper range of flexibility and motion without tightness and pain. There must be a balance of strength from the front of the body to the back and comes to the side as well as from top to bottom.

The hip flexors that include the gluteus muscle group and the iliopsoas muscle group must be able to keep the body in peak performance condition. When looking at the power location of the body, it's situated in the very centre. Though both legs and arms are important, they cannot be compared to the importance of hips as real power rests on hips.

It is not possible to twist, jump as high as far, dive or run without powerful hips. Essentially it is not possible to stand a chance of being an athlete when the hips are having health problems. Another area for the athletes to consider on the issue of hips is during their preparation for play. Most often they need to lean forward whether lining for a race or picking up a ball, and it must be in a forward position.

These athletes don't stand in a casual, upright position as this position will not be able to generate enough power to gain the needed momentum.

To make a move, the feet should be wide apart, knees flexed, and the torso by leaning forward. This position will prepare the athletes for whatever happens, as he is balanced in the best possible to launch quickly. Professional's athletes understand the importance of hips flexors and the power it carries to raise their performance. It doesn't matter if they know the chemistry behind it, but they are taking steps to improve overall physical and mental health.

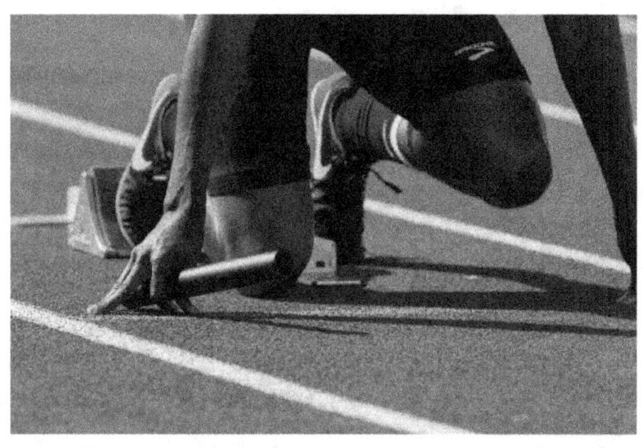

There is this happiness after performing certain physical activity. You feel energize and achieve emotional boost, whenever you walk a little, perform certain physical labour, or complete an exercise. This boost includes the release of endorphins. When the body is moving, there will be released of production of stress-relieving hormones. Don't forget that the human body is designed to move throughout the day. We are not meant to sit all day. Having regular workout will not only improve physical health but also in feeling better and be more energetic.

Take care of your Hip flexors

It is not compulsory to be an athlete to focus on your health. The fact is that everyone should be concerned about their physical well-being. It is your sole responsibility to understand how to improve the performance of your hip flexors. Though work to be done to improve the health of your hip flexors does not come easy, but you will need to put in some hard work. It requires your commitment, not just a few exercises or stands up and conclude that it's better.

Remember, as discussed earlier, that hip flexors are the most important muscles for hip flexion, which means that hip flexors are critical for moving the leg forward. The gluteus Maximus (glutes) are needed to extend hip that will move the leg back. The muscles required are situated high on the hips and can control the femur bone. And when these muscles are in proper shape and balance, it's an indication that you possess adequate glute activation.

However, if the hip flexors are weak, then the muscles situated further down on the hip and thigh will have to carry out the majority of the work. This is an indication that other muscles are compensating for the lack of strength in the hip flexors; thereby leading to many health issues such as lower back pain.

When the above problem is not treated, it may lead to a posterior pelvic posture. A posterior pelvic position happens when the hip flexors and glutes are not well activated. Instead, it is the TFL and hamstring muscles that will be developed, that will make the head of the femur to slide out partially from the socket, creating a hip pain.

This condition occurs when you sit for too long. Another reason is when the hip flexors tighten, and the butt is stick out, so they prevent the gluten from functioning properly. This will lead to a kind of posture where the butt will stick out too far. When this situation happens, it leads to a kind of pain and problems that are similar to a problem associated with posterior pelvic posture. Note that tight hip flexors may cause back pain and hamstring strains. But this is preferred to weak hip flexors.

To improve the glute activation patterns, you may need to work on the muscles that are attached to the higher part on the hip. These are the muscles expected to control movement, rather than those attached on the lower part of the hip. The muscles that connect to the thighbone is to keep the head of the femur tight in the hip socket. When this fit is not comfortable, there will be glute activation problems. What we are trying to drive at is that many people are suffering from non-existent glutes because of sitting too much or not doing a great deal on their glutes.

When the glutes refused to perform as expected, there will be a problem that resulted from reduced hip strength. The two problems associated with this issue are overshadowed glutes and inhibited glutes.

Inhibited Glutes:

A condition where the glutes failed to contract properly will lead to inhibited glutes. This condition is very common to those that sit all day and can affect anyone, even including athletes. People that cannot walk, stand, or move, have their glutes not working properly.

This can be as a result of many problems like injury or posture.

Overshadowed Glutes:

This happens when the glute is working properly but are not as strong as other muscles in the lower body region. Such condition will occur when the quadriceps and adductor groups are more developed than the glutes. This situation will make the body to go on compensation by relying on other muscle groups. The effect of this is that when the body required to compensate with other muscles, the balance will be thrown off and will lead to additional complications, such as chronic pain. An activity such as sprint that is explosive where the most influential muscle groups will handle the majority of the work. So having overshadowed glutes will make you have more power in your things than the glutes.

Effects of Psoas Muscles on the Glutes

Weak psoas muscles may lead to inhibited glutes and overshadowed glutes. A situation of forcing other muscle groups to overcompensate lead to overshadow glutes, while sitting all day will result from inhibiting hip flexors, psoas and glutes.

The solution to glutes issues is to restore the balance. The step is to lose the hip flexors and also strengthening the glutes and help in increasing hip mobility. This will lead to a reduction in lower back pain and will also improve performance in sports and everyday activities.

EFFECTS OF TIGHT HIPS ON WEIGHT

We have discussed that psoas is very involved in the fight or flight response of the body. This response makes you to either attack or retreat when in danger. In as much that psoas is very involved in the physical and emotional reactions, a tightened psoas will always signal to your body that you are in danger.

The moment the body is in danger the SNS (sympathetic Nervous System) will activate the body's natural survival instinct that will use up the adrenal glands, depleting the immune system in as much as the body assumed dangerous situations. Unfortunately, tight hips will send biofeedback similar to the assumed danger to the brain. When such feedback is sent from the hips to the mind, the body will remain in that survival state.

Don't forget that the human body is designed in such a way to survive, and also has a natural response to protect itself from what may happen or when facing dangerous conditions. The body would want to curl up like a ball to protect its vital organs.

Imagine if the physical body is always in a curl position, just like the way we sit in a chair, the mind will always respond to body position as if it is in danger. In other words, if you sit all day, the hips will short, pulling you into the fetal position. It is this fetal position that the brain relates to survival.

Now let consider how this affects our state of survival. With the situation explained above the adrenal glands will become overworked and will be exhausted later. The adrenal gland is responsible for our response to stress, by secreting hormones that are related to the stress levels. These hormones will control hormonal cycles and functions in the body. The moment adrenal glands are overworked, the body will prepare for danger by storing fats and calories.

Among other health issues that adrenal imbalance can cause include an expanded waistline. This is how it pans out. Naturally, when we are hungry, our blood sugar will drop, and the brain will send a signal to the adrenal glands to release cortisol. It is the duty of the cortisol to activate fats, glucose, and amino acids so to keep our body fueled with energy till we eat.

Cortisol helps in the maintenance of blood sugar levels, insulin, and in assisting the cells in absorbing glucose. When faced with long time stress like sitting for all day, both cortisol and insulin will remain elevated in the blood, and the extra glucose will be stored as fat in the abdomen.

What frustrates about the storage is that they are not necessary and will be in the abdominal area and thighs. What we can't exclude is that physiological responses happen whether real or fake. The real problem is that most of the stresses we face daily like sitting, do not require the actual fight or flight response. So we open our body to engage in what we don't need to do. And since there is no imminent danger when we sit all day in a chair, we don't need the extra calories the body is storing in preparation for survival.

Effect on overall health

Psoas is considered as the most important muscles in the body. And disregarding this truth is the beginning of foolishness. We all want to live healthy and happy, but we become stuck in our normal routines without making changes. Not that they are all bad, but it becomes terrible routines when it includes unhealthy habits.

How Tight Psoas makes you fat

Do you know that having tight hips may make you look a little fat?

Have you seen a skinny person and yet possess a potbelly stomach?

The main reason a skinny person could have potbelly stomach is when he is having the poor posture that may be as a result of a tight psoas. When the tight psoas is having an issue with belly, it is an issue of space rather than a fat problem. An overweight problem will always be and feel like a fat, but space will look and feel differently. Fat is known to be soft and plump, but when the cause is the psoas, your spine comes out of alignment, thereby forcing the abdomen to come out forward. A stomach with a potbelly that occurs as a result of tight hips will have no fat, will be reasonably hard, and somewhat rigid.

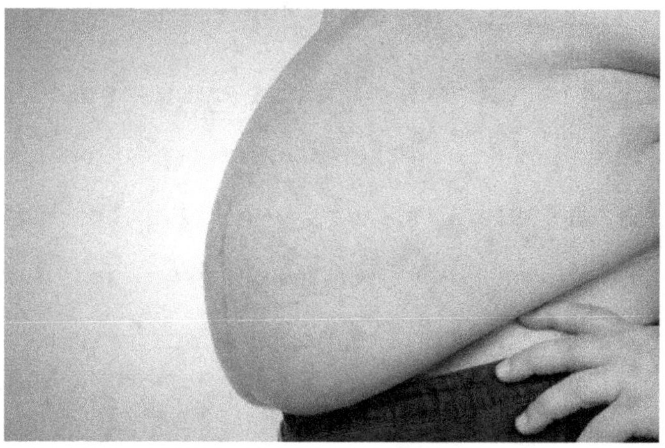

So the issue is how does psoas cause pot belly?

The psoas is so designed that it attaches from the legs to the spine via a connection from the back of the inner thigh and along the lower portion of the spine. A perfect spine will move down from the spine and curls around the back of the pelvis before reaching its way forward to the down and back to attach to the inner thigh bone. It is a known fact that the majority of organs and muscles comfortably are in front of the psoas and can easily be shifted when there is a stress or movement is done.

But when the psoas is being compromised by sitting all day, and there is no work -out on the hips, the anterior pelvic will tilt. This condition will lead to belly been popped out from the forward tilting of the pelvis. A tight psoas is known to pull forward off the back of the pelvis and shift everything in front of it. This shifting includes both small and large intestines. No wonder that with this condition psoas will affect digestion in a colossal way.

This happens as a result of both or one of the psoas is tight. The rule is, the tighter the psoas, the more pressure will be placed on organs and other muscles. This will lead to unwanted changes in the body functions and also on a restriction in the physical movement.

It is important to know if your anterior pelvic tilt or if the tilt is what is normal for your body.

A certain measure of tilt is reasonable in human, and it has been discovered that women tend to have more tilt than men. To know the actual degree is to know the actual shape of your spine.

If you want to know the degree of anterior pelvic tilt, take off your shirt and stand sideways in the mirror. You will see one of the three reflections:

1. You are fat and no way around it.

2. You are thin but having a curved spine with a potbelly.

3. You look balanced and normal.

It is easy to see how you look if you are suffering from tight hips. However, this is not the only yardstick to know tightness. It is possible to have good posture but still having psoas tightness. So the earlier experiment is not the final diagnosis, but it will show you how your abdomen and spine line up.

EFFECTS OF WEAK PSOAS MUSCLES ON EMOTION AND ENERGY

Impact of Weak Psoas Muscles on Emotion and Energy should not be underestimated.

Have you discovered that if you spend the whole day in a chair, you tend to be more tired than when you spend the whole day on physical activities? This reason is not farfetched as it is partially due to the effect of psoas muscles. Don't forget that a tightened psoas muscle will prevent you from letting go of stress accumulated on a day. Instead, it builds and builds stress every day.

You can let go of your daily stress by learning how to relax the psoas muscles. If you can do this, you will be able to boost your emotional health. Don't forget that psoas muscles are not only required for stability and balance, but it has other functions more these two. The psoas muscles are directly connected to emotions and our natural survival conditions.

The way the human body expresses various emotions is different from the way other animals does. As this depends on the condition of psoas muscles, as the more relaxed the psoas, the better relaxed you will be. It does more than stability as said earlier. The psoas muscles connect to the deepest survival instincts. It will ground you to the immediate surroundings.

When stressed, angry or afraid, all these emotions are travel through the nerves in the psoas muscles, via the spine and to the brain. In a nutshell psoas, muscles act as messengers.

They are messengers as they relay emotions and information to the brain. So logically, when the psoas muscles are healthy, then the feelings that will be getting to the brain will be without distortion, as there will be greater clarity in the communication process. However, if the psoas is in an unhealthy state, the communication will be distorted or cramped.

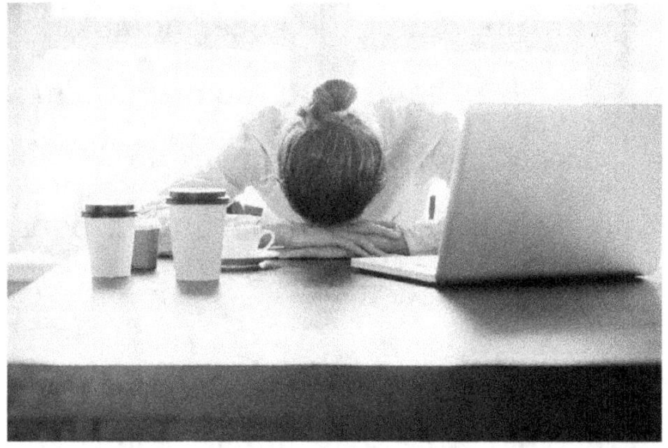

Do you know that the discomfort you have after a long day sitting in a chair is more connected to the psoas muscle than the stress coming from the work? Physical stress worsened the mental stress, that why it leads to more physical stress. When the psoas muscle is relaxed, you will be more relaxed and less discomfort. This invariably applies to physical and mental health.

Though there are real pains associated with a tight psoas muscle -pains that may lead to hip and back pain, others are knee and ankle pain. The psoas also connects to the diaphragm, and this is used for breathing. This is an indication that not only is psoas connected to response to fight or flight, and it's also connected to the ability to breath.

With the ability of psoas muscles connecting to several functions in the body, it shows that psoas muscle is a central force in the overall health.

Remember when your psoas muscles are healthy, your emotions will freely travel from the spine to the brain. You will not be blocked mentally by tight psoas muscle, and you will be able to think more clearly throughout the day.

Never have you allowed fear to dominate your life. Start with focusing on your psoas muscles and other hip flexors. If you can unlock your hip flexors, it will help you in overcoming mental or physical stress that may want to get on your way.

Steps presented later in this guide will help in improving your strength and mobility; it will guide you in developing your emotions. The results will be the ability to be creative, calmer, more grounded and ready to face any daily challenges.

STRETCHING

Stretching is known to be a form of physical exercise for a specific tendon or muscle or group of muscles to be deliberately stretched or flexed for it to be improved in elasticity and to achieve a comfortable muscle tone. The expected result is a feeling of increase muscle control, full range of motion, and flexibility. Also, stretching can be used to correct and alleviate cramps and be able to improve the functions in daily activities by increasing the range of motion.

Stretching has been known to be a natural instinctive activity as humans and animals perform it, and most times it is accompanied by yawning. Most times, it occurs immediately after waking up from sleep, after coming out of confirmed spaces, or after the end of the day physical activities.

Several incidents and studies have shown that stretching can be dangerous when they are performed wrongly. We have several methods for stretching, but most are dependent on which muscle or group of muscles to be targeted. Some stretching techniques have been known to be detrimental to the point of leading to instability, hypermobility, permanent damage to muscles, tendons, or ligaments.

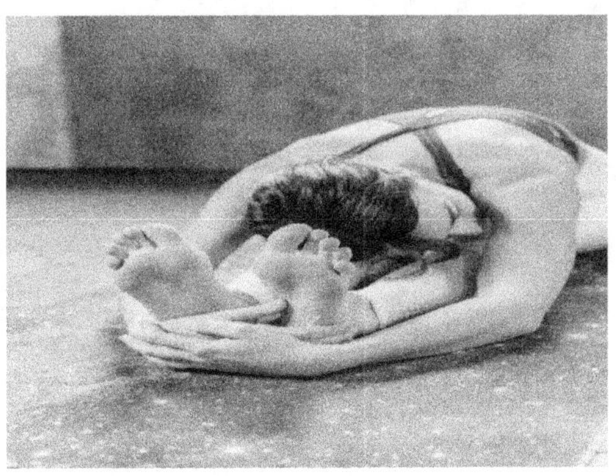

Types of Stretching

We all familiar with static stretching, where we hold a stretch for a certain period, and then we release it. But there are many other types of stretching that include passive, dynamic, and active stretching. All the stretching techniques mentioned below are not as static as they are meant for specific applications and additional advantages.

Static Stretch

Static stretching is the type of stretching that is common, and people are doing it on a regular basis. The Massachusetts Institute of Technology (MIT) stated that static stretching includes stretching the muscle or group of muscles to its limit and then be able to maintain the stretch. An example includes seated hamstring stretch; in this method, the goal is to reach the toes and hold it between 15 to 30 seconds.

There were reports and debates about when the static stretching is efficient. A report from the Scandinavian Journal of Medicine & Science in Sports in March 2013, stated that the static stretch before a workout might be detrimental to reducing strength, performance, explosiveness and power. However, recent research from Frontiers in Physiology in November 2019, reported that short-duration static stretching does either part or alone of a full warm-up work out has little effects on performance.

Dynamic Stretching

This is a type of stretching recommended to be before a workout rather than using static stretching. The dynamic stretching is used to control movements that are expected to bring muscles to its maximum range of motion gradually. The dynamic stretching includes jump, squats, leg swings, and high kicks.

All the above methods will help in stretching muscles and increase blood flow, and a great addition to any exercise. But remember to warm up with some light cardio before engaging in dynamic stretched.

Select dynamic stretches that are meant for a particular activity, if you want to work on the lower back, choose high kicks or leg swings, provided is upper body, select shoulder mobility with towel or dowel, or arm swings.

Active Stretching

Active stretching is similar to static stretching, as it depends on antagonist muscles and agonist muscles (quadriceps and hamstrings). Active stretching is expected to make use of the strength of an agonist muscle that will hold the body in a position to stretch the antagonist muscle and can be kept for a particular time. An example of active stretching is bringing a leg up in front as high as it can be held thereby making use of strength in the leg. The agonist muscles (hip flexors, and quads) contract, making the hamstrings and glutes relaxed and release in a kind of way called reciprocal inhibition. In yoga, an example of active stretching is a wide-legged seated forward fold.

Ballistic Stretching

This type of stretching makes use of momentum to force a limb above its normal range of motion. This practice is done by bouncing in and out of position- like swinging leg up to a bar with force at a height that is very uncomfortable to reach to movement. According to MIT, ballistic stretching is dangerous to the general population as it doesn't allow the muscles to relax and adjust to the expected stretched position. It will make them tighten up due to stretch reflex, and this reflex is a protective measure by the body to guard against muscle been over-stretched.

Passive Stretching

Some people mix passive stretching with static stretching. Though they are similar, there are differences in them. Passive, also known as relaxed stretching as it acts to relax the muscle as much as possible while stretching.

While in the passive stretch, it is vital to take a position and maintain it by making use of another part of the body, a partner, apparatus to hold. An example of passive stretching can be seen when raising a leg and holding the back of the thigh with hands.

Isometric Stretching

According to MIT, isometric stretching is very effective than active and passive stretching. As the isometric stretching makes use of the resistance of other muscle groups and contractions of the muscles to be stretched.

The work behind the isometric stretching is complicated, but MIT made us understand that if a muscle is already stretched before contractions are held in the position for a long time, the initial passive stretch overcomes the stretch reflex, thereby triggering muscle lengthening.

You have the liberty of doing isometric on your own or with the help of a partner. Those you can do alone include holding on to the ball of the foot, then make use of calf to try to straighten the instep for the toes to be pointed. An example of the one with a partner can be seen when you lie on the back with a straight leg in the air, and your partner pushes your leg to you while you are trying to resist it. Hold the position for 8 to 15 seconds, and then relax the leg for 20 seconds before starting another set.

PNF Stretching

Proprioceptive neuromuscular facilitation (PNF), according to MIT, is not a kind of stretching but a way to combine isometric and passive stretching. It is expected that PNF will result in maximum static flexibility. PFN was originally developed for stroke patients.

PNF requires you to have a partner that will provide resistance against an isometric contraction and be able to move to joint passively through its more massive range of motion. Few everyday uses of PNF technique are hold-relax, where the muscle is isometrically contracted for 7-15 seconds. The muscle will be allowed to relax for a few seconds before been subjected to passive stretch that will stretch the muscle more than the initial stretch.

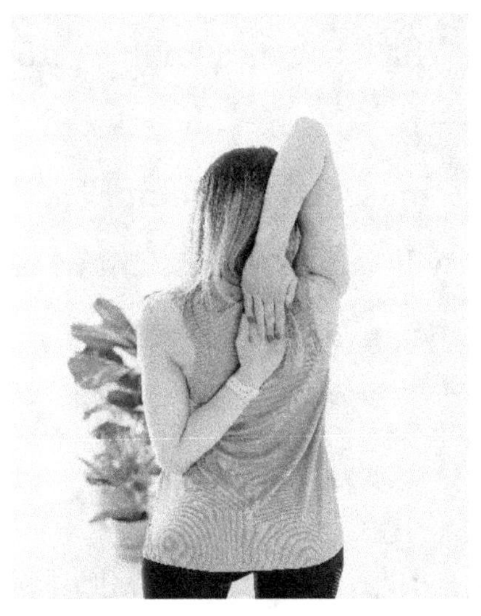

Benefits of Stretching

Stretching has been known to offer many benefits to body and mind. Adding stretching into the daily routine will make the muscles to be well circulated and healthier. Some of the benefits of stretching are discussed below:

Benefits of stretching for the body:

Flexibility

Stretching has been known to improve flexibility. The more you stretch, the more flexibility muscles become. With time, stretching will later become more comfortable for the body, invariably resulting in improved flexibility.

Posture

Stretching will improve posture. Poor posture can easily be reversed and healed while undergoing daily stretching. Stretching will strengthen muscles and enhances proper alignment, thereby making the body posture more vertical.

Prevention of injury

As you prepare your muscles for different exercising movements, the more your likelihood of having an injury is reduced. When the muscles are warm and stretched, body movements become easier, thereby helps when preventing injury.

Increases Nutrients and Reduces Soreness

Stretching increases the blood supply and also increases the amount of nutrients to muscles. This happens as a result that stretching will allow the blood to circulate through the body, and the nutrients in the blood will be circulated and spread throughout the body. As the nutrients increases and blood increases, there will be a reduction in the soreness.

Advantages of stretching for the mind:

Calming of mind

Stretching every day will offer the mind a mental break. It will allow the body to recharge the blood flow throughout the body, thereby resulting in a calmer and peaceful mindset.

Tension released

Many people carry stress in their muscles. When having the feeling that is overwhelmed, the muscles tighten and will act as a defensive strategy. The more the stretch, the less tense muscle will be. Note that stretching is a good way of stress management.

Increase Energy

Due to the fact that stretching allows an

increased in blood and nutrient pass through the body. The body feel refreshed, and the energy levels will be increased.

Tips on stretching

It is advisable to understand the proper stretching technique. It is crucial you are stretching correctly so to prevent injury. Remember that improper stretching can lead to muscles been damaged. Do not overwork when you are injured or already having a tense muscle. While stretching and you are feeling pain, it is better to ease up on the strained muscle to prevent damaging the muscle even more.

When stretching focus more on significant muscle tendon, and are hips, legs, neck, upper back, lower back, shoulders, and pelvis. Remember always to do your stretching routine daily. As the more you stretch, the more benefits your body and mind will receive.

STATIC STRETCHING, NOT THE ONLY ANSWER

Understanding what tight hip flexors is one thing, knowing what to do to solve the issue is a different ball game.

Many YouTube videos suggested that holding a few static stretches for a certain period will get the job done. Or rolling with a tennis ball stuck to the hips will remove the health issues.

In all honesty, it's not only a tennis ball and foam roller that will get your hip flexors in shape. And if you are not careful, they may even damage the hips more. The main reason why it is hard to fix the hip flexors is due to the fact that it is hard to reach the area. The psoas muscles are buried deep inside the core of the human body, making it hard to access. No wonder it needed more than just a simple static hip flexor stretch to unlock it.

Have you discovered that most of the stretches you are doing are having a minimal effect? It's because you have to attack the psoas muscles from differed angles making use of various exercises methods to unlock the muscles in the right way. The bare truth is you can do it all by yourself if you know how to unlock it. Take it just like a safe lock that requires a set of several numbers to unlock it. Once you are with the correct numbers, the safe is yours to be controlled.

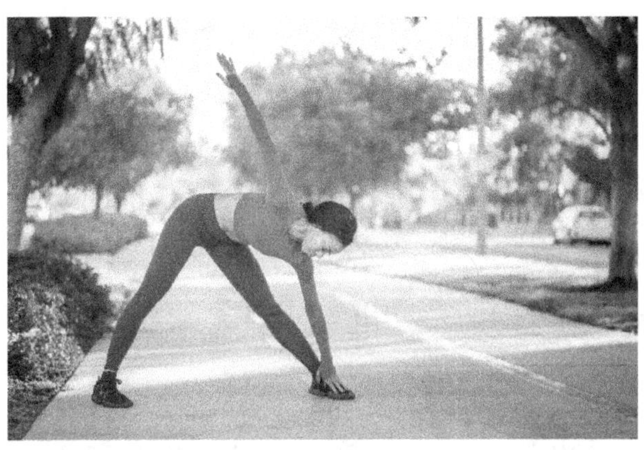

There are specific movements that go beyond the static stretching and can be employed to unlock and loosen the hips, back and legs. Some of them are;

Dynamic Stretching: With this stretch, you will be activating the muscle around a joint and moving the joint via its full range of motion in a progressive manner. This will lead to an increased range of motion around the joint, thereby warming up the muscle around the joint and help in improving circulation around the joint. This is just like butt kicks or high knees.

PNF Stretching: PNF is also known as proprioceptive neuromuscular facilitation. This is a method where you will be activating a particular muscle for it to relax the muscle around a joint, to decrease the stiffness around a joint.

Mobility Exercises: Mobility exercise will target the joint, movements and exercise that will help the joint to function excellently. This technique makes the joint to move freely.

3- Dimensional Core Stability Exercises: This technique is used to target the muscle in all planes of movement for the core and abdominal muscles to have good activation, strength, and endurance that may lead to a decrease in unnecessary stress that may damage joints.

Muscle Activation Movements: Many of our muscles are not working properly as a result of sitting all day. You can use the technique to target those muscles that are off and keep working properly so to make the body move efficiently.

Fascia Stretching: This technique will target the tissue that muscles surround and start exercising on loosening and lengthening the fascia.

Now you the right technique to unlock the hip flexors, but the vital question of how you combine them to give the best result.

THE POWERFUL HIP FLEXORS DIET

Leg Swings

Steps:

1. Stand on a block that is raised an inch or two off the ground.

2. Hold something for support, such as ledge, door, or wall (optional)

3. Swing your leg in a total of three different directions to target a complete range; perform the complete series in 5 times total.

4. Stand on either block or pad with one foot. Swing the opposite leg forward and backward;

perform the complete set in 5 times total.

5. Next step is to swing the leg sideways in 5 times.

6. Swing leg at a 45-degree angle for 5 different times in each direction.

7. After you have observed the above steps, then switch to the opposite leg and repeat the steps in 5 times.

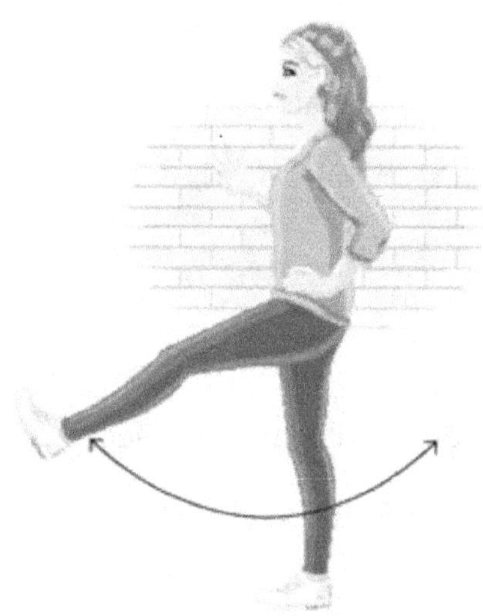

Leg Swing

Quad Stretch

Steps:

1. Use the right hand to grab the top of your right foot.

2. Pull the heels to your butt. You will feel a slight stretch in front of thighs.

3. Increase the intensity of the stretch by bulling knee backward a little further and make sure you keep the abdominal area tight.

4. Stretch the opposite arm straight up toward the ceiling (optional).

5. Hold the stretch for 20 seconds and then repeat the steps with the other leg to complete one cycle.

6. Perform 2 total repetitions.

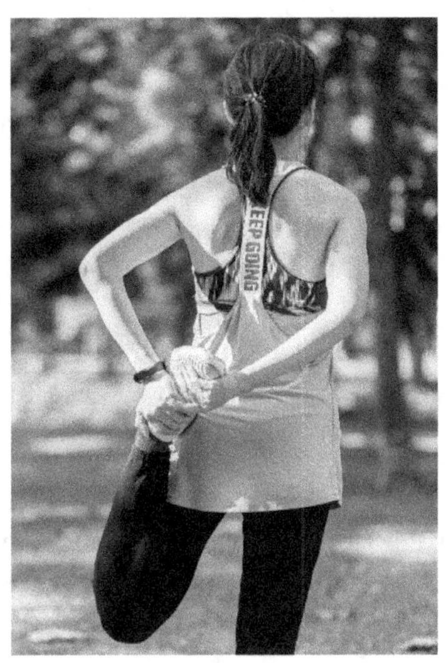

Quad Stretch

90/90 Kneeling Stretch

Steps:

1. Keep your legs at 90-degree positions with one foot flat to the ground. Make sure the opposite knee is resting on the ground.

2. Let your knee, hips, and ankle are in 90-degree positions.

3. Let your back flattens to the ground so to increase the intensity of the stretch.

4. Tight the abdominal muscles and raise your arms overhead.

5. Make sure to contract the glutes so to bring your hips forward.

6. You will experience a little stretch in front of the thigh.

7. Hold the stretch for 20 seconds and repeat for the opposite leg.

8. Repeat the steps twice on each side.

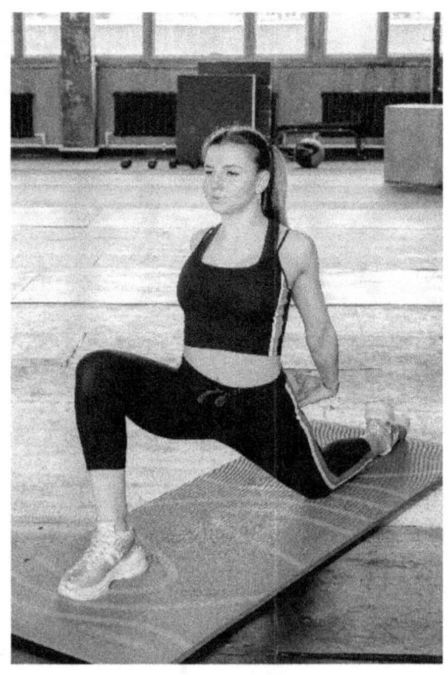

90/90 Kneeling Stretch

TABLE HIP FLEXOR STRETCH (FASCIA STRETCHING)

This technique is similar to squad stretch

Steps:

1. Stand with your back very close to the bench.

2. Hold the right foot with the left hand.

3. Pull the heel toward the back.

4. Stretch the right arm toward the ceiling. Rest the heel on the bench as you pull it back.

5. Use the bench to stretch yourself further, and you should feel a slight stretch through arms, abdominal muscles, and knee.

6. Bring the knee further out to increase the intensity of the stretch (optional).

7. Hold this step for 20 seconds and do the steps twice with each leg.

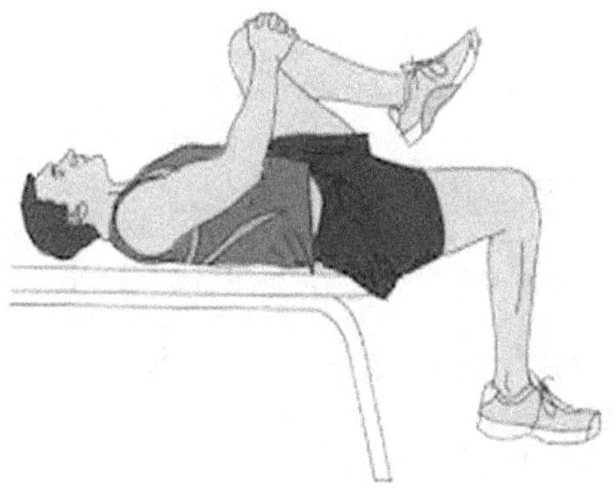

Table Hip Flexor Stretch

HIP AND BACK EXTENSION

Steps:

1. Launch into a kneeling position and place the hands on the hips.

2. make sure you arch backward and hold it for two seconds before getting to the start position.

3. Do these steps 5 times.

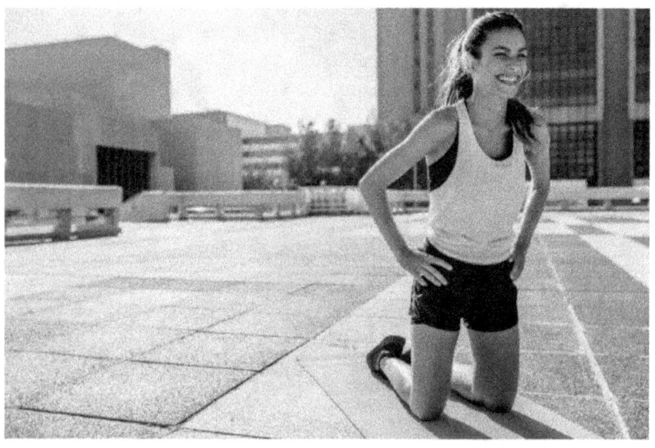

Hip and Back Extension

Laying on Back with Knees Out and In

Steps:

1. Lie on the back, keep the knees bent, and make sure your feet are flat on the ground.

2. The feet should be hip-width apart.

3. Let your arms be at a 45-degree angle to your sides.

4. Lower the knees to one side, back to the starting position, and back to the other side, then return to the starting position again.

5. Hold the position for 2 seconds each time you lower the knees.

6. Do these steps for 5 times.

4-Point Hip Back into Hip Exercises

Steps:

1. First make sure your knees are hip-width apart.

2. Rock the hips back and concentrate on the movement of hips and not the back.

3. Once the lower back starts to curl, separate the knees further. Make sure you keep the back straight while rocking.

4. Once only the hips move, come back to a kneeling position.

5. Rock the hips for 5 times and hold each side for 2 seconds.

6. Rock the hips at an angle for three different cycles in an arch direction.

7. Hold each cycle for 2 seconds on each side.

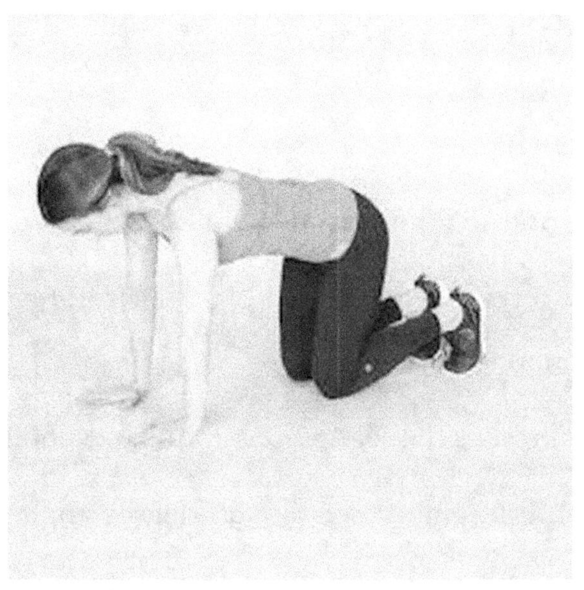

4-Point Hip Back into Hip Exercises

Heel into Wall

Steps:

1. Lie on the floor next to a wall.

2. Lie on the stomach and place the forehead on your hands.

3. Make sure the legs are extended out behind.

4. Bend the right knee to a 90-degree angle.

5. Rest the outside of the right foot on the wall.

6. Push the outer part of the foot into the wall with slight force with the aid of hip muscle.

7. Hold this position for 6 seconds, and then do it again.

Do it 6 times and then switch legs.

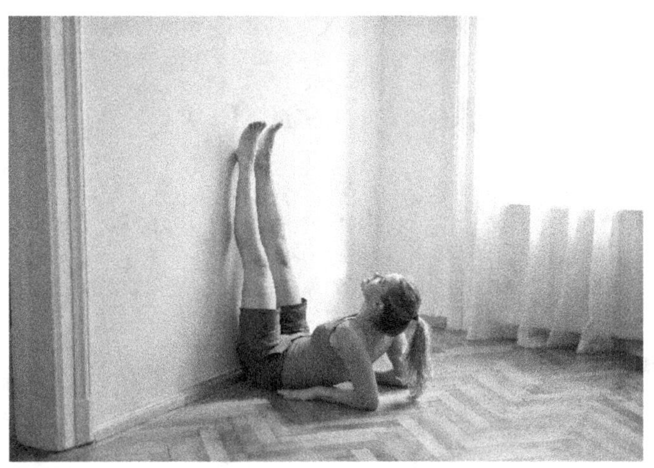

Heel into Wall

FRONT TO SIDE PLANK

This technique is a 3-dimensional core stability work out. It is a front plank position technique.

Steps:

1. Be on good alignment.

2. Rest the upper body on the forearms.

3. Pose a straight line from the shoulders to the ankles.

4. Once in an aligned position, roll to one side.

5. Make sure you roll into a side plank pose.

6. Bring leg upward to keep the spine straight in this movement.

7. Hold this position for 2 seconds

8. Get back to the front plank position, roll to the other side, and then hold the position for two seconds.

9. Do these steps for 5 times.

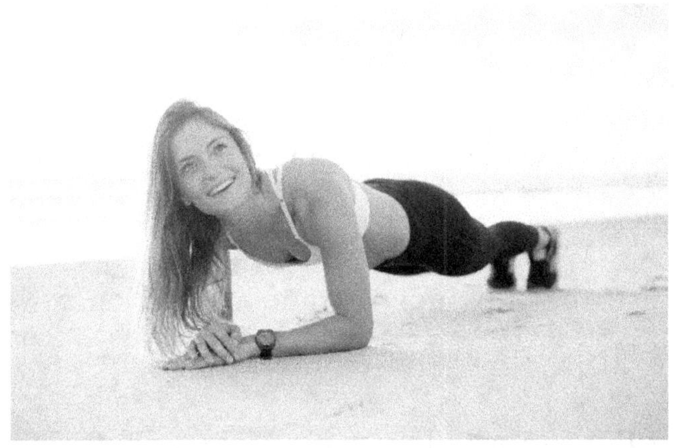

Front to Side Plank

Single-Leg Gluteus Bridge

This is the final stretch to unlock your tight hip flexors.

Steps:

1. Lie on the back and brace the abdominal muscles.

2. Raise the hips upward and extend one leg forward.

3. Let the opposite leg bent while straightening the raised leg, and then hold this position for 2 seconds.

4. Lower the leg in the air and bring it to the starting position.

5. Do the steps with the other leg.

6. Hold the position for each cycle for 2 seconds before getting back to the starting position.

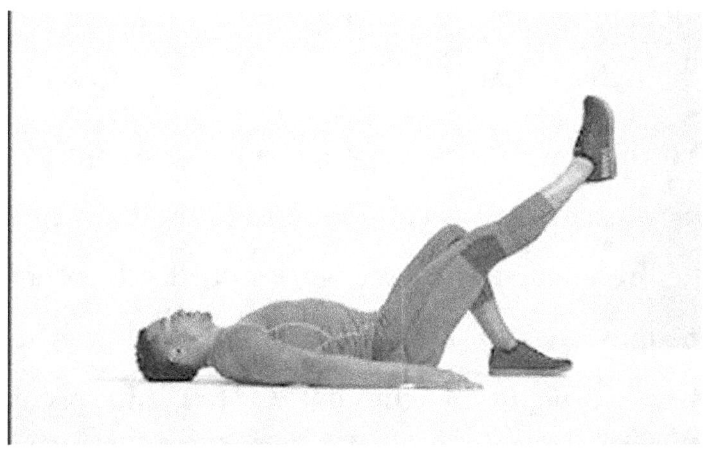

Single-Leg Gluteus Bridge

Start these stretches NOW

The above routine covers 10 stretches that should be your daily routine. They give a complete solution to unlock your hip flexors. With these work out your hip flexors will start loosening and lengthening and also psoas muscle will benefit from it.

The stretches will take only 20 minutes to complete. It is advisable to perform these techniques, not less than 5 times a week to get the best results.

To those who have experienced severe injuries, or muscle strains should consult their doctors before engaging in new work out. But to other people, these exercises are the perfect way to start focusing on the hip flexors and psoas muscles. Just make a commitment to perform the stretches daily.

HIP FLEXOR STRETCHES FOR ELDERS

Experience and studies have shown that seniors tend to experience more of hip flexor pain when compared to younger adults as a result of the older you get, the weaker the muscles. When the pain in the hips is escalating, it becomes a daunting issue to do a simple task without experiencing uncomfortable.

TIGHT HIP FLEXORS IN SENIORS

As we are ageing there comes some health issues that may include hips and hip pain. It is known that people over the age of 60 tend to be ten times more likely to have pain and discomfort in their hips as a result of osteoporosis and other underlining health conditions.

As discussed before, hip flexors help when it comes to walking, running, bending over, and some other daily task that is taken for granted. The muscles or group of muscle that make up the hip flexors include, the psoas, iliacus, Sartorius, femoris, and iliocapsularis.

When any or more of the muscles mentioned above become weak or strained, it will lead to tightness and pain in the hips. This tightness and pain may cause sharp pain in other parts of the body, such as the lower back.

HIP FLEXOR STRETCHES FOR ELDERLY

The following hip flexor stretches for seniors are designed to unlock their hip flexors and keep it flexible. And if impressive results are to be achieved all the below stretches must be carried out regularly to attain mobility, reduction of pain, and strengthening of muscles of hip flexor.

SEATED HIP FLEXOR STRETCH

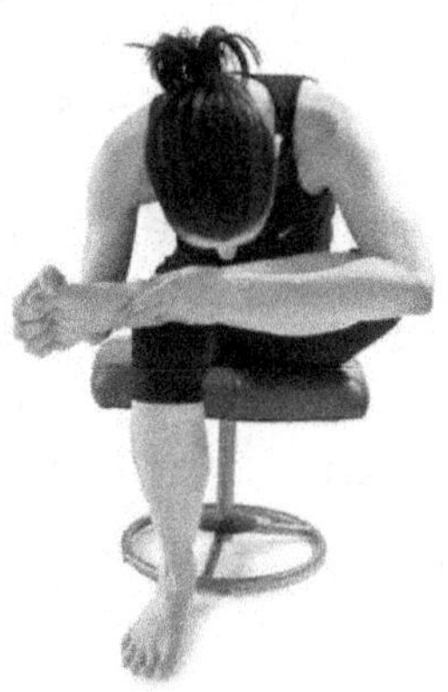

Seated hip flexor stretch is a great mobility exercises on hips for the elderly as it will help in stretching the main flexor muscles and enhances the reduction of tightness.

Observe the following steps when undergoing the seated hip flexor stretch.

Steps:

1. Get a chair and sit on it.

2. Place yourself at the edge of the chair.

3. Bend your knees in a 90- degree angle and make your feet wholly planted flat on the ground so to push your hips to the left.

4. Push your hips to the left side of the chair as you hold your left side.

5. Lean your body on the chair till the upper back is touching the head of the chair.

6. Next, hold your left foot with the left hand and raise it behind the chair. (If it is difficult to stretch the left foot behind the chair as far as you can go).

7. Allow the left foot in this position behind the chair for a minimum of 10 seconds and then release it.

8. Return the left foot to the starting position.

9. Repeat the whole steps by switching to the right foot.

Butterfly Stretch

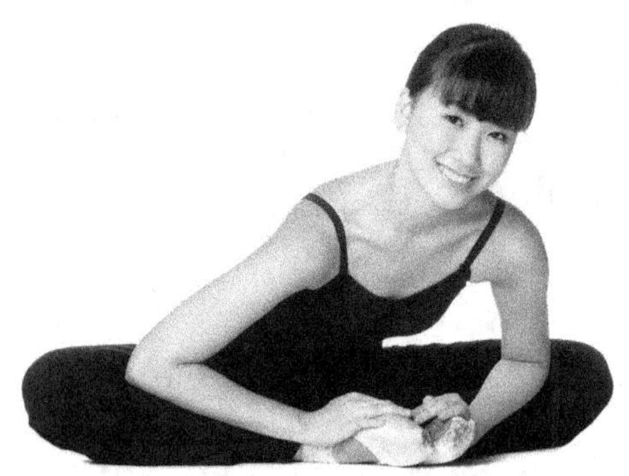

This stretch is excellent for the elderly when experiencing tight hip flexors, as it reduces the hip pain and maintains the hips mobility.

Steps:

1. Sit flat on the floor with your legs bend at your sides.

2. Make sure the soles of the feet are touching each other when in this seated position.

3. Place your hands on each of your ankles in front and lean forward as far as you can go.

4. Make sure you use elbows to push down on your knees hanging at sides slightly.

5. Hold this position as you push the knees with your elbows for 15 seconds.

6. Return to the starting position after 15 seconds.

PIGEON POSE

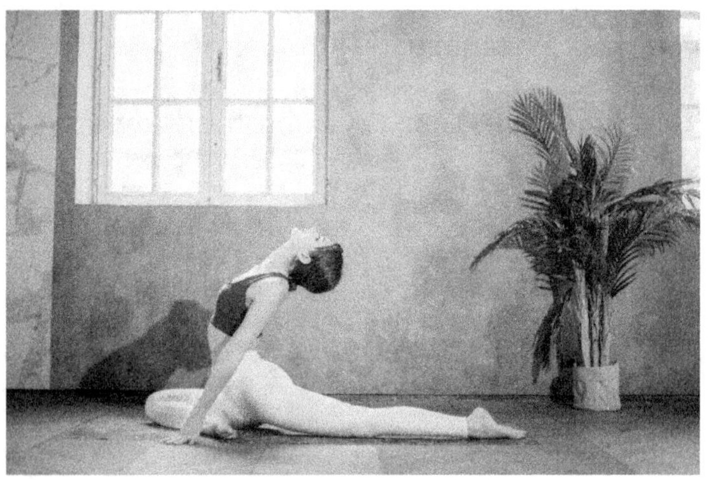

This stretch is easy and great for the elderly having tight hip flexors, as it will improve hip mobility, and helps in the alleviation of tight hip flexors symptoms.

Steps:

1. Get down on the hands and feet as if to go on pushups.

2. While in this position, push your right knee forward and right behind the right hand.

3. Make sure to fold the upper portion of your body over the right leg while the left leg will be in a straight position behind you.

4. Hold onto this position for 15 seconds.

5. Then return to the push-up position you started.

6. Repeat the steps by switching to the right knee with the left knee.

FIGURE FOUR STRETCH

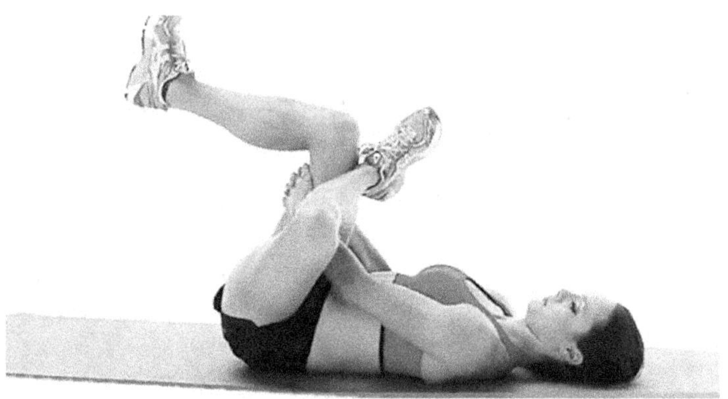

Figure Four Stretch is one of the best hip mobility exercises for the elderly as it will help in stretching the main flexor muscles and enhances the reduction of tightness.

Observe the following steps when undergoing the stretches known as seated hip flexor.

Steps:

1. Lie on your back, and while lying, make sure

to bend your knees and keep the feet flat against the floor.

2. Move your right ankles and place it on top of the left knee.

3. Use your hands to hold your left leg and pull it up toward the chest area.

4. Hold this position for a minimum of 15 seconds and return to the starting position.

Note: When you feel the burn in hips and glutes, it means you are doing the stretches correctly.

TIPS FOR THE ELDERLY TO PREVENT TIGHT HIP FLEXORS

It is crucial for the elderly to know that the only way to avoid the pain associated with hip flexor muscles is to be active every day. The more they

stay active like moving around, the less likely is
for their hips flexors getting short, becoming
tight, and leading to pain.

CONCLUSION

I'm happy that you have made it to the end of this guide. We have covered some groundbreaking chapters that have to do with your health. The information dished out was created to teach you the functions of hip flexor and its responsibilities for your emotional health, stability, and general well-being.

It is not funny how most people do not realize that psoas muscle is one of the essential muscles in the human body. It is the duty and function of this muscle to keep us upright, and in connecting the upper part of the body to the lower part of the body.

As discussed in the previous chapters, the effects of spending a large part of your life sitting in a chair are putting pressure on the psoas muscle. As with time, the muscle will start to shorten, tighten, and will lead to back pain and other health-related issues.

To correct these health issues, this guide offers some combination of exercises and hips movement that will stretch your muscles and put your psoas under relaxation.

Don't forget that if your work requires you to sit all day, always get up every 30 minutes to prevent tight hip flexors. Just get up from the chair, walk, take a break to relax your body and perform some light form of stretches before sitting again.

Remember sitting in a chair for 6 to 8 hours every day will lead to a severe impact on your overall health.

Now, it is time to put into practice all that you have read. Get up and start the stretches, as illustrated in the previous chapter.

Thanks for reading.

References

Journal of Education and Training Studies: "Effect of Ballistic Warm-Up on Isokinetic Strength, Balance, Agility, Flexibility and Speed in Elite Freestyle Wrestlers"

Massachusetts Institute of Technology: "Physiology of Stretching"

Pacific College of Health and Science: "Thai Massage Can Open Joints, Stretch Muscles, and Rejuvenate Energy"

https://www.livestrong.com/article/539154-7-types-of-stretching-exercises